Getting P/her/sonal: A Self-Discovery Wellness Journal for Women

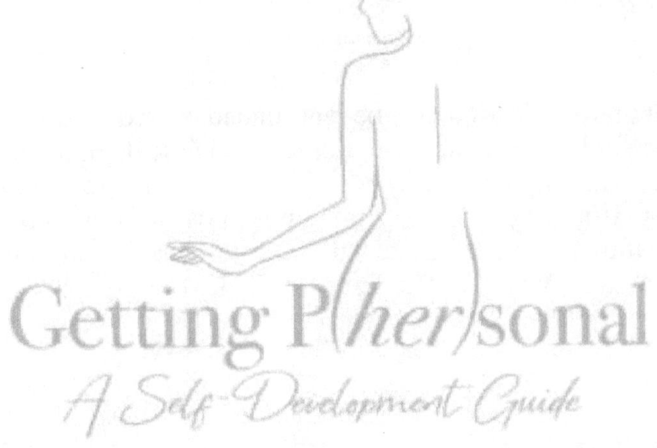

A Self-Development guide focusing on Personalized self-care through holistic health

Muna Yvette Ezumah-Ezekwo, B.S, M.S, MPH

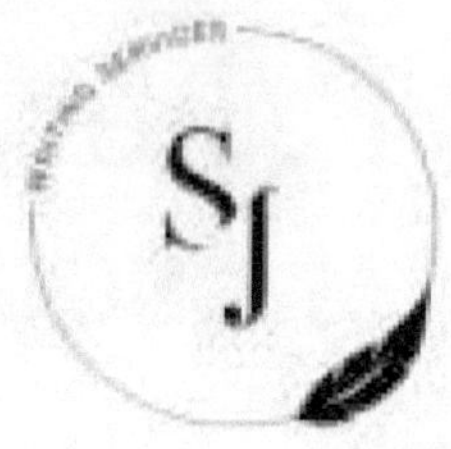

SJ Writing Services LLC
Publishing
Columbia, South Carolina

First Edition
Copyright 2026 by Muna Yvette Ezumah Ezekwo
All rights reserved.

Table of Contents

Introduction

We often talk about building ourselves for the future, whether it's searching for our forever home, launching a new business, or simply starting a workout or nutrition routine to feel "summer ready." In every area of life, we're constantly looking for what's next, what's better, and what truly works for us so we can thrive rather than just survive. Yet, finding the perfect routine or guide isn't always easy. It requires us to set the tone, become the true investigators of our own lives, and be intentional about shaping our present to make space for what's ahead.

We are here because we're ready to begin. Starting a journey of self-development and fulfillment opens the door to becoming our most aligned selves. And there is no better time than now to explore the "how," "what," and "when" of our growth, allowing our minds, bodies, and whole selves to transition into a more grounded, purposeful way of living. Through self-work, we cultivate self-worth, and through self-worth, we build the foundation for the life we've always envisioned.

There are so many internet "self-taught coaches, gurus, and experts" claiming to know the best way for us to live, often competing with one another about who has the right formula, the right information, or the perfect approach. We search through countless communities, hoping to find that one clear path to becoming our ideal selves. But if we're honest, no one truly offers a personalized guide that shows us how to begin cultivating our optimal selves across our careers, relationships, health, and personal growth.

So how do we discover who we really are? How do we understand our own likes, dislikes, needs, desires, passions, and purpose in a way that helps us reach our goals and build a healthy life from the inside out? Each of us carries unique values that contribute to our individual growth. The real journey is learning what fits you, not what works for the masses.

What may look like just another prompted journal is actually a vessel, an intentional space for self-work, where you can practice your aspirations, align your motivation, and develop the habits, mindset, and actions that support a healthier, more grounded lifestyle. Personal health and well-being must be prioritized because caring for our mental and physical bodies becomes the foundation upon which all other goals are built. That means making conscious choices about our nutrition, staying active, getting restorative sleep, managing stress, and surrounding ourselves with supportive, meaningful relationships.

We all share the desire to show up as our best selves, whether you identify with an active, holistic, nomadic, urban, or digital on-the-go lifestyle. A holistic approach to self-care allows us to enhance our overall functioning and maintain a sense of balance. This might include setting intentional goals, creating action plans across different areas of life, and checking in with ourselves regularly. Just as important is recognizing how our daily choices shape our health; unhealthy routines like poor nutrition, excessive alcohol, drug use, or chronic stress can significantly impact our physical and mental well-being. Choosing differently, even in small ways, can transform how we feel and how we move through the world.

Now that we've brought our goals and intentions into the open, what better place to start than with the basics? Let's explore what happens when we become our own investigator, cheerleader, teacher, and source of joy. Let's step into our own consciousness and discover connections we never realized were there. Let's learn how to be guided by truth, alignment, and intention.

Come on! Let's Get P/her/sonal.

Dedication

To my mom, the most beautiful and God-fearing woman I know, thank you for being my foundation, my example, and my strength.

Getting Started

We'll tap into ourselves through our lifestyle, but first, let's see what makes us... us. Our hormones love to remind us that they're running the show. They lift us up during the highs, tug us down during the lows, and sprinkle emotions everywhere in between. When they're happy, life flows. When they're not... well, they make sure we know. Our diets join the party too, and our bodies respond to every food group, every strange new ingredient, and sometimes even our own inner thoughts. Think of it like studying for a test: if we don't prepare for things like the flu, high cholesterol, or maintaining good gut vibes, we can't expect top-tier "results." And the gut? Oh, it sends the loudest signals of all. We can't ignore them, just listen, assess, and give it what it needs at the moment. After all, it's trying to help us get where we want to go. When we talk about hormones, chronic disease prevention, diet, sleep, stress, basically all the fun parts of being human, the real goal is figuring out what to welcome into our lives and what to kindly show the exit. There's always space to explore what we <u>want</u> while staying true to what we <u>need</u>. Sometimes our wants will win, and that's okay. Just know that the best benefits tend to show up when we're ready for them. Health, physical, mental, emotional, and everything in between is worth prioritizing, no matter where you are on your journey. My hope is that this guide meets you exactly where growth is calling. So let's walk this path together. Let's keep evolving, learning, and building the kind of generational health literacy that sticks.

You've officially got a place to turn when you need gentle guidance and a little encouragement along the way. So everyone.... "Get Started!"

Block 1: Self-Work & Personal Growth

Self-work, Self-love, Self-worth: the trifecta of "thriving" energy. It's all about learning how to nurture ourselves spiritually, physically, and mentally while calling in a healthier, happier lifestyle. This is where we start embodying everything we're meant to feel: grounded, aligned, and a little bit magical.

Be proud of your journey, every twist, pause, breakthrough, and "wait... what am I doing?" moment. Growth isn't supposed to be perfect; it's supposed to be yours. So sprinkle self-compassion everywhere you go. You deserve it just as much as the life you're manifesting.

Self-Work Toward Self-Worth

When you wake up each morning,
what pops into your mind first?

"What's for breakfast?"
"Do I have meetings today?"
"Can I squeeze in the gym?"

Our brains sprint before our feet even touch the ground, sorting through hundreds of thoughts and choosing the loudest ones to start the day. And we rarely question it, we call it "routine," a normal way to begin the morning. But tucked in between those practical questions are tiny, sneaky stressors that slip in before we've even had a chance to breathe. Over time, mornings like this can quietly create more tension than peace. What we often forget is that taking just a moment, one intentional pause, can shift us from frantic to purposeful. The world is already full of noise; there's no need to invite it into the few sacred, silent moments you still have to yourself.

So starting tomorrow, try this: give yourself <u>30 uninterrupted seconds</u> of meditative quiet as soon as you wake up. Whether the sun gently wakes you or your alarm blasts you into reality, take those 30 seconds anyway. Notice the difference in how you move through the day. Let this become a small ritual that begins your larger journey of self-work, a journey that leads to genuine self-worth.

In a perfect world, working on ourselves would be smooth and effortless. No setbacks, no comparison spirals, no emotional plot twists. But real life is... real. We fall short sometimes. We get discouraged. We pause progress. And still, each day we return to work because deep down we know we are worthy of more than worry, anxiety, and fear. New challenges will come, and with them the chance to rise. Self-work is the key to unlocking the version of self-worth that aligns with a healthier, more fulfilling lifestyle.

Morning Routine and Grounding Moments

- ♥ Mineral water with lemon and lime or green tea (supports hydration and antioxidant intake)

- ♥ Chasteberry (supports menstrual cycle regulation and may reduce PMS symptoms)

- ♥ Bone broth (supports gut health and provides essential nutrients)

- ♥ A blood-sugar-balanced breakfast within 45-60 minutes of waking

- ♥ Gentle movement such as yoga, stretching, or a short walk

- ♥ Deep breathing or a brief meditation practice

- ♥ Pause for five slow, intentional breaths to calm your nervous system and support your body's natural detox flow

You don't need to do everything, choose 2–3 habits that feel supportive and build from there.

Building Healthy Habits

You may be wondering how all this ties together. Self-work and self-worth move hand in hand; one is the cause, the other is the effect. When we commit to doing the work, we naturally begin to see shifts in our bodies, our habits, and our emotional landscape. We gain clarity around our triggers, our patterns, and the behaviors that drain us or throw our hormones off balance. As we unravel these patterns, we can build both daily and long-term habits that shape a new, empowered beginning. This journey is especially important for women, whose hormones often signal imbalance before our minds even catch up. By understanding the biological connection between emotions and physical health, we can honor our bodies with compassion instead of frustration. Throughout this guide, my goal is to give you the tools to nurture your holistic well-being, mentally, physically, emotionally, and spiritually. Be proud of your journey, your process, and your progress. And above all, treat yourself with care. Self-compassion is part of the work, too.

Why You Feel Low Energy

No one wants to start the day dragging their feet. Your morning energy sets the tone for everything, meetings, conversations, errands, and even that one email that somehow ruins your mood for three hours.

Low energy can often be traced back to root causes like:

- Skipping breakfast or inconsistent eating patterns

- Dehydration

- Chronic stress or dysregulated cortisol levels

- ♥ Nutrient deficiencies (like iron, B vitamins, magnesium)

- ♥ Poor sleep quality or insufficient rest

- ♥ Thyroid imbalances

- ♥ Unmanaged stress

- ♥ Inconsistent use of supportive supplements

Low energy usually isn't random, it's your body trying to tell you something.

Simple solutions to boost energy:

- ♥ Balance your blood sugar throughout the day

- ♥ Eat enough protein early in the day

- ♥ Choose gentle caffeine options (such as green tea)

- ♥ Consider magnesium and B-complex vitamins (as needed)

- ♥ Support gut health with prebiotics and probiotics

- ♥ Manage stress with intention

- ♥ Improve your sleep habits

- ♥ Limit screen time and bright lights at least 30 minutes before bedtime

Big Sister Guidance: Starting the Journey
Women, Hormones & Balance

Our hormones often reflect what our bodies are experiencing long before we put it into words. Supporting hormone balance is essential, not only for fertility, but for overall health and well-being.

Key areas that matter:

- ♥ Estrogen balance and its role in reproductive health

- ♥ Cholesterol's role in hormone production

- ♥ The connection between hormone imbalances and fertility

- ♥ Nutrition strategies that support progesterone balance

- ♥ A hormone-supportive diet that nourishes the whole body

Your hormones are not your enemy; they're messengers. When we learn to support them, everything from mood to metabolism to mental clarity begins to shift.

Pause & Reflect

Take a moment here. There's no right answer.

If your current routine reflects what you believe you deserve... what is your routine saying about you?

Getting P(her)sonal

A Self-Development Guide

Getting P(her)sonal

A Self-Development Guide

Getting P(her)sonal

A Self-Development Guide

Getting P(her)sonal

A Self-Development Guide

Getting P(*her*)sonal

A Self-Development Guide

Getting P(her)sonal

A Self-Development Guide

Getting P(her)sonal

A Self Development Guide

Getting P(her)sonal

A Self-Development Guide

Getting P(her)sonal

A Self-Development Guide

Getting P(her)sonal

A Self-Development Guide

Getting P(her)sonal

A Self-Development Guide

Getting P(*her*)sonal

A Self-Development Guide

Getting P(her)sonal

A Self-Development Guide

Block 2: Hormone Balance and Function

Our bodies are incredible storytellers, and hormones are the little messengers that narrate the plot. They shape our energy, mood, digestion, sleep, stress responses, motivation, and even how glowing our skin decides to be on any given Tuesday. I used to think something was wrong with me when my energy, mood, and body felt inconsistent. It wasn't until I understood hormones that everything started to make sense. When they're in balance, everything feels smoother. When they're not... well, they make their imbalance loud and clear. Let's break down the main characters of this hormonal universe, light-heartedly, but with a real understanding of how they keep our bodies moving.

Estrogen: The Architect of the First Half

Estrogen is one of the body's primary female sex hormones, and it plays a powerful, multifaceted role. Produced mainly by the ovaries (with support from the adrenal glands and fat tissue), estrogen helps regulate the menstrual cycle and supports several key functions, including:

- Building and thickening the uterine lining

- Maturing the egg leading up to ovulation

- Supporting mood, bone health, and skin elasticity

Estrogen is most active during the first half of the menstrual cycle, the follicular phase, where it prepares the body for ovulation. After ovulation, progesterone becomes the dominant hormone, and estrogen steps back as the cycle transitions into its next phase. If pregnancy does not occur, hormone levels shift, the uterine lining sheds, and the cycle begins again. It's a beautifully coordinated process, one guided by the balance between estrogen and progesterone.

Low Estrogen: What It Can Feel Like

When estrogen levels drop, your body usually lets you know, sometimes subtly, sometimes more clearly.

You might notice irregular or shorter cycles, low energy, mood swings, anxiety, sleep disturbances, low libido, or brain fog. Sometimes, it simply feels like something is "off," even if you can't fully explain it. Low estrogen is often connected to how supported your body feels overall. When the body is under-fueled, under chronic stress, or lacking consistency in daily habits, estrogen levels can be affected. This is why the focus isn't on doing more, it's on doing the basics well. Start with nourishment. Make sure you're eating enough and eating consistently. Balanced meals that include protein, healthy fats, and carbohydrates help stabilize your system and support hormone production. Movement should feel supportive and strengthening, not exhausting. Sleep should be protected, and stress should be managed with care, not ignored. Estrogen also plays an important role in maintaining bone density and overall long-term health. As levels decline, especially over time, bone loss can accelerate, which is why consistent nutrition and strength-based movement become even more important for long-term support (Riggs, Khosla, & Melton, 2002).

Estrogen responds to stability.

When your body feels safe, nourished, and supported, it becomes much easier for your hormones to find their rhythm again.

When estrogen levels drop, your body usually gives subtle, and sometimes not-so-subtle, signals.

You might notice:

- ♥ Irregular or shorter cycles

- ♥ Spotting between periods

- ♥ Low energy or persistent fatigue

- ♥ Mood swings, anxiety, or irritability

- ♥ Sleep disturbances

- ♥ Low libido

- ♥ Brain fog or difficulty concentrating

When the body is in a constant state of "go mode," it may deprioritize reproductive hormones.

Gentle practices like breathwork, journaling, time outdoors, or simply slowing down can help restore that balance. When your body feels safe, nourished, and supported, it becomes much easier for your hormones to find their rhythm again.

Progesterone: The Calming Counterpart

Progesterone is often called the relaxing hormone, and honestly, she deserves the title. Produced after ovulation by the corpus luteum (the temporary structure that forms after the egg is released), progesterone dominates the second half of the cycle, the luteal phase.

Progesterone plays an important role in the body by helping to:

- ♥ Helps balance the effects of estrogen
- ♥ Supports healthy sleep patterns

♥ Prepares and maintains the uterine lining

♥ Supports early pregnancy

♥ Plays a role in regulating mood

If pregnancy does not occur, progesterone levels drop, the uterine lining sheds, and the cycle resets. When progesterone is low, you may feel it, PMS, mood swings, fatigue, heavier periods, or heightened anxiety. But when it's balanced, everything feels steadier, calmer, and more like yourself.

Low Progesterone: What It Can Feel Like

When progesterone levels are low, the body often feels it more clearly, especially in the second half of the cycle.

You might notice:

♥ PMS symptoms

♥ Anxiety or mood fluctuations

♥ Heavier or irregular periods

♥ Fatigue or low energy

♥ Increased abdominal weight

♥ Hair thinning or shedding

♥ Difficulty with fertility

You may also feel more emotionally reactive, less grounded, or as though your body is struggling to find balance.

Progesterone is deeply connected to how safe and supported your body feels. When the body is under chronic stress, undernourished, overexercised, or sleep-deprived, it may prioritize survival over hormone balance. Focus on steadiness: balanced meals that include healthy fats and protein, stable blood sugar, consistent sleep, and intentional stress support. These signals help your body feel safe, something progesterone depends on. Also focus on vitamins B, C, and D, along with zinc, support hormone synthesis, immune balance, and ovarian function. Supporting these through whole foods, and supplementation when appropriate, can help restore balance. Blood sugar stability is equally important. Meals that combine protein, healthy fats, and fiber help regulate energy and support a more stable hormonal response. Stress support is key. Practices such as journaling, therapy, breathwork, prayer, or intentional rest help signal safety to the body, something progesterone depends on. Sleep is another major factor.

Without adequate rest, hormone regulation becomes more difficult, and symptoms may intensify. Thyroid health also plays a role. Because the thyroid and reproductive hormones are closely connected, supporting thyroid function through nutrition, stress management, and medical care when needed can indirectly support progesterone balance (Mullur, Liu, & Brent, 2014).

Progesterone responds to calm and consistency.

When your body feels safe, rested, and supported, it becomes easier for your hormones to stabilize.

The Hormone Cycles Explained
Hormones As Messengers

Hormones are tiny, invisible messengers traveling through your bloodstream, delivering instructions throughout the body, like overachieving interns carrying important messages.

They are the language your body uses to communicate with itself, sending subtle signals that keep every system connected and working together behind the scenes (Hall & Hall, 2021). They turn food into energy, keep your breathing steady, and help your body repair and renew. They decide when you're sleepy, when you're stressed, when you're growing, and when your reproductive system wants to have a meeting. They also have strong opinions about your mood, sometimes sharpening your focus, sometimes making you cry at a commercial.

In many ways, hormones are the quiet conductors of your internal orchestra, unseen but powerful, making sure everything stays in rhythm... even if they occasionally throw in a dramatic solo. Their rhythms follow daily cycles (circadian) and monthly cycles, and when those rhythms are disrupted, everything from energy to emotions can feel off-beat (Leproult & Van Cauter, 2010).

Testosterone: Not Just a "Male" Hormone

Testosterone matters for women too, more than we often realize.

When levels are low, you might notice:

- ♥ Low libido

- ♥ Increased abdominal fat

- ♥ Fatigue

- ♥ Emotional ups & downs

- ♥ Difficulty losing weight

- ♥ Hair thinning

- ♥ Weakness or reduced muscle tone

- ♥ Irregular cycles

Often overlooked, testosterone plays a key role in energy, strength, mood, and metabolic health in women.

If your testosterone feels low, the answer isn't to push harder; it's to support your body more intentionally. Hormones thrive on nourishment and rhythm. Begin by making sure you are eating enough, especially quality protein and balanced meals that include healthy fats. Your body needs a consistent supply of fuel to produce and regulate hormones effectively. Undereating or chronic restriction can quietly disrupt that balance. Move in ways that build strength and vitality. Strength training paired with moderate cardio can support resilience and energy. The goal is not exhaustion, it's steady, empowering movement that leaves you feeling strong. Stress management is equally important. When your nervous system remains in a constant state of stress, hormone balance can shift (Chrousos, 2009). Create simple daily rituals to support regulation, quiet mornings, breathwork, sunlight, journaling, and intentional rest. Small moments of calm add up over time. Protect your sleep. Seven-nine hours of restorative rest allows your body to recover and recalibrate. Hormonal health is built during recovery, not constant activity. If appropriate for you, gentle support such as maca powder or a consistent supplement routine may offer additional support. Balanced testosterone isn't about intensity; it's about creating an internal environment that feels nourished, steady, and strong.

Daily Habits that Affect Hormones

When hormones are in harmony, the difference is noticeable. Energy becomes steady instead of unpredictable. Stress feels more manageable rather than overwhelming. PMS softens, moods stabilize, and sleep becomes deeper and more restorative. Cycles feel more regular and less painful. Skin appears clearer, hydration improves, and even daily routines feel lighter and more enjoyable. There is often a quiet return of joy, not dramatic, but steady.

Hormonal balance does not happen by accident. Emotional, physical, environmental, and stress-related triggers all influence how your hormones respond. Once you begin to recognize these patterns, you can shift your habits in ways that support long-term stability rather than constant fluctuation. Certain daily patterns can quietly disrupt this balance. Poor sleep, excessive caffeine, overworking (even from home), too much cardio without recovery, perfectionism, restrictive eating, skipped meals, chronic stress, and weak boundaries all place ongoing pressure on the body. These habits may feel normal, or even productive, but over time, they drain energy and challenge the nervous system. When this happens, your body begins to signal for support. Fatigue may set in, immunity may weaken, and symptoms such as headaches or joint discomfort may appear. Sleep may become inconsistent, appetite may fluctuate, and emotional overwhelm may feel closer to the surface. These are not failures; they are signals. Your body is asking for balance, not more restriction or pressure.

In contrast, supportive daily habits create a sense of steadiness. Balanced digestion, hydrated skin, regular ovulatory cycles, stable energy, consistent mood, deep sleep, and strong immune function are all signs that your body feels supported. These outcomes are not built through extremes, but through rhythm, nourishment, rest, and aligned routines. When one area improves, others often follow.

Long-term wellness is less about dramatic changes and more about daily consistency. When your habits communicate safety and stability, your hormones respond with balance.

How Hormone Balance Transforms Your Life

We've just stepped into the world of hormonal harmony, where your choices, habits, emotions, biology, and lifestyle come together to tell a deeper story. This chapter marks the beginning of building a healthier, more aligned version of yourself.

My intention is to create a safe, reflective space where you can explore your habits, shift your patterns, and make sustainable changes that feel supportive rather than forced. Holistic wellness is about honoring the whole person, mind, body, emotions, and spirit. When all four are supported, a more balanced and meaningful path toward healing and long-term transformation begins to unfold.

How to Make These Habits a Lifestyle

- ♥ Get to know yourself deeply

- ♥ Check in with yourself daily

- ♥ Set boundaries that protect your peace
- ♥ Feel your emotions without judgment

- ♥ Use your voice with confidence

- ♥ Release relationships and environments that no longer support you

- ♥ Spend intentional time with yourself and listen inward

Remember, finding what works for your body is a journey, not a race. Every hormone, habit, and lifestyle shift responds differently from person to person, and that is completely okay. Think of yourself as an observer in your own life, gently testing, learning, and adjusting along the way. Approach this process with patience and self-compassion. What supports someone else may not be your perfect fit, and that does not make your progress any less meaningful. Consider this big-sister guidance: I am here to support you, not to pressure you. Everything shared here is grounded in both lived experience and scientific understanding, so you can move forward with confidence and care. To anchor this conversation in science, the role of hormones in regulating energy, mood, sleep, and reproductive health is well established in endocrinology research. Hormones function as chemical messengers that travel through the bloodstream, coordinating communication between organs and tissues and helping regulate metabolism, stress responses, reproduction, and circadian rhythms (Hall & Hall, 2021).

Research also shows that reproductive hormones, such as estrogen and progesterone, interact closely with neural systems involved in mood, sleep, and emotional regulation (Baker & Driver, 2007). These hormones naturally fluctuate across the menstrual cycle and can influence sleep quality, cognition, and emotional stability.

For example, estrogen plays a role in neurotransmitter systems related to mood and stress, while progesterone metabolites interact with GABA receptors in the brain and may contribute to calming and sleep-supportive effects. Hormonal rhythms are also closely tied to circadian patterns and lifestyle factors, including sleep, stress, nutrition, and light exposure. When these rhythms are disrupted, changes can occur in metabolic function, emotional regulation, and reproductive signaling (Leproult & Van Cauter, 2010). In other words, the "rhythm" discussed throughout this chapter is not just a metaphor; it is biological.

The endocrine and nervous systems work together as an interconnected network that continuously responds to your internal and external environment. When your body receives consistent signals of nourishment, rest, movement, and stress support, these systems are better able to function efficiently and maintain long-term balance.

Pause & Reflect

Take a moment here, Take a breath, and respond.

"If your body could send you one clear message right now... what would it say?"

Getting P(her)sonal

A Self-Development Guide

Getting P(her)sonal

A Self-Development Guide

Getting P(her)sonal

A Self-Development Guide

Getting P(her)sonal

A Self-Development Guide

Getting P(*her*)sonal

A Self-Development Guide

Getting P(her)sonal

A Self Development Guide

Getting P(*her*)sonal

A Self-Development Guide

Getting P(her)sonal

A Self-Development Guide

Getting P(her)sonal

A Self-Development Guide

Getting P(her)sonal

A Self-Development Guide

Getting P(her)sonal

A Self-Development Guide

Getting P(her)sonal

A Self-Development Guide

Getting P(her)sonal

A Self-Development Guide

Block 3: Nutrition For Hormone Health

Nutrition with Intention

Hormonal changes affect how your body processes nutrients, stores energy, and regulates appetite. Signs of hormonal imbalance, such as weight changes, irregular cycles, hair loss, mood shifts, fatigue, digestive issues, or persistent skin concerns, are often early signals that something within us needs more support.

Because women move through distinct hormonal phases across the lifespan, our nutritional needs are not just important; they are foundational. Food is not simply fuel; it is information. It communicates directly with our hormones, shaping how we feel, function, and heal. As we move toward a more personalized approach to health, understanding these differences allows us to align our eating habits with our biology. Instead of working against the body, we begin to nourish it in ways that feel supportive, intentional, and sustainable.

Why Consistent Eating Matters

A balanced and consistent eating pattern supports both metabolic health and hormonal rhythm (Jakubowicz et al., 2015). When meals are skipped or spaced too far apart, the body shifts into a state of stress and uncertainty. Over time, this can disrupt blood sugar regulation, energy levels, and hormone signaling.

In contrast, nourishing the body with regular, balanced meals, especially those rich in whole, minimally processed foods, creates stability. With consistency, the body often responds with:

- ♥ Smoother digestion

- ♥ More stable blood sugar

- ♥ Steadier energy and mood

- ♥ Improved appetite regulation

- ♥ Stronger cellular repair and recovery

Whole foods play a key role in this process. They slow digestion, deliver more nutrients per bite, and support the body's natural ability to maintain hormonal balance (Aune et al., 2017). Over time, these small, consistent choices create a foundation of internal stability.

Nutrition Needs Shift Across Life Stages

The female body is not static; it evolves through seasons. Puberty, pregnancy, postpartum, perimenopause, and menopause each bring meaningful hormonal transitions that influence metabolism, body composition, and emotional well-being. As hormones shift, so do nutritional needs. For example, during menopause, declining estrogen levels can influence fat distribution, often leading to increased storage around the abdomen (Santoro et al., 2021). This is not simply a result of aging. Estrogen plays a critical role in metabolic regulation, and as levels decline, the body adapts accordingly. These changes may also affect cardiovascular health and long-term weight regulation. Understanding these differences allows us to personalize how we eat. When we recognize that hormonal transitions influence how the body processes nutrients, stores energy, and regulates appetite, we can begin to adjust our nutrition with intention.

This showed up for me as trying to "eat healthy" but still feeling tired and off. Once I focused on balance instead of restriction, my body responded completely differently. Instead of resisting change, we learn to work with the body. Awareness allows us to make choices that feel supportive rather than restrictive, creating a more sustainable and compassionate approach to nourishment

Gut Health: The Foundation of Hormonal Balance

The gut is often overlooked in conversations about hormones, yet it plays a central role in overall hormonal health. Beyond digestion, the gut influences inflammation, immune function, and even mood regulation. A well-supported gut can help regulate estrogen metabolism, reduce systemic inflammation, and strengthen overall endocrine function. For the gut to function optimally, its internal ecosystem must remain balanced. This includes maintaining a healthy ratio of beneficial to harmful bacteria, supporting digestion through balanced meals, and consistently consuming adequate protein, typically around 20–30 grams of protein per meal, an amount shown to support tissue repair, muscle maintenance, and overall metabolic stability (Phillips, 2014).

Prebiotic- and probiotic-rich foods further support this balance (Gibson et al., 2017). Foods such as kiwi, yogurt, kombucha, onions, and garlic provide beneficial bacteria or the fibers that nourish them. In some cases, targeted supplementation may also be helpful. When gut health is supported, hormonal balance often follows. A well-functioning gut contributes to clearer thinking, more stable moods, improved digestion, and stronger immune resilience. In many ways, caring for your gut is one of the quiet but powerful foundations of hormonal harmony.

Blood Sugar Balance: The Hormone Stabilizer

Stable blood sugar is one of the quiet foundations of hormonal balance (Ludwig et al., 2018). When blood sugar remains steady, energy feels consistent rather than unpredictable. Emotional stability improves because rapid glucose swings no longer amplify stress responses. Sleep often becomes deeper and more restorative, as nighttime cortisol disruptions are reduced. Hormones such as insulin, cortisol, and progesterone function more smoothly, and even hunger cues become clearer and more reliable. Small, intentional shifts in nutrition can create meaningful change. Pairing Greek yogurt with berries and a spoonful of nut butter combines protein, fiber, and healthy fats to slow glucose absorption. Adding protein powder to baked goods can transform a quick carbohydrate snack into a more balanced, sustaining option. Swapping refined pasta for zucchini noodles, chickpea pasta, or lentil pasta increases both fiber and protein intake, further supporting stability.

These changes may seem simple, but over time they reinforce hormonal balance. Consistency, not perfection, is what allows the body to regulate, recover, and thrive.

Thyroid & Hormones: Supporting Your Metabolism

The thyroid plays a central role in regulating metabolism and how the body uses energy (Mullur, Liu, & Brent, 2014). When thyroid function is disrupted, the effects can extend beyond metabolism, influencing energy levels, mood, digestion, weight, and even other hormone systems. Because the thyroid works closely with reproductive and stress hormones, imbalance in one area often affects the others. Supporting thyroid health begins with a few key foundations. A well-functioning gut is essential for proper nutrient absorption, which directly impacts thyroid activity (Thursby & Juge, 2017). Nutrients such as iodine, selenium, and zinc are especially important, as they are required for the production and activation of thyroid hormones. Certain herbs, including ashwagandha, astragalus, maca, and American ginseng, may also provide gentle support when used appropriately. Equally important is reducing inflammation and managing stress. Chronic stress can interfere with thyroid hormone production and utilization. The gut, brain, and thyroid are deeply interconnected, often referred to as the gut-brain-thyroid axis (Mayer et al., 2015). When digestion, stress, and nutrition are supported together, thyroid function is more likely to stabilize.

Hormonal balance is rarely about correcting a single system. It is about supporting the body as a whole so that everything can function in alignment.

The Hormone Balance Framework

No single food or supplement creates lasting change. What matters most is what you do consistently. Hormonal health is built on a few foundational patterns that, when practiced regularly, allow the body to function at its best.

First, protein. Adequate protein intake helps regulate appetite, supports skin health, and stabilizes hormones. When protein needs are met, cravings tend to decrease, and energy becomes more consistent.

Second, blood sugar balance. Unbalanced meals can lead to energy spikes and crashes, contributing to fatigue, cravings, and even skin concerns. Pairing carbohydrates with protein, fiber, and healthy fats helps maintain stability throughout the day.

Third, inflammation. The goal is not restriction, but nourishment. A diet rich in healthy fats, antioxidants, and whole foods supports the body, while minimizing excess sugar and heavily processed foods helps reduce internal stress.

Fourth, micronutrients. Often overlooked, these play a critical role in hormonal health. Nutrients such as magnesium, zinc, and iron influence energy, skin, and metabolic function. A varied, whole-food-based diet helps meet these needs naturally. When these foundations are consistent, the body begins to respond. Energy stabilizes, digestion improves, and skin often reflects that internal balance.

That "glow" people talk about isn't created—it's revealed. It's what happens when your body is consistently supported.

Mindful Eating: Learning to Listen to Your Body

Many of us have become used to eating while distracted, scrolling on our phones, working, or watching something in the background. Over time, this disconnect makes it harder to recognize when we are truly satisfied.

And satisfaction is not the same as fullness. You can feel physically full and still crave more if your meal did not provide what your body actually needed. This is where balance becomes essential. Meals that include protein, fiber, and healthy fats help regulate hunger signals, allowing you to feel both satisfied and sustained. Without that balance, your body continues to ask for more. When supported with fiber, resistant starch, and fermented foods, it communicates more effectively with the brain, helping regulate appetite and satiety. Mindful eating is not about control; it is about awareness. It is about paying attention, honoring your body's signals, and giving it what it truly needs.

"Satisfaction comes from balance, not from eating more."

Portion Balance:

Understanding What Your Body Needs

Portion control often gets misunderstood. Too much food can leave you feeling heavy and fatigued, while too little can lead to cravings, low energy, and instability. True balance lies in giving your body the right amount of nourishment. A well-balanced meal includes protein, carbohydrates, healthy fats, and vegetables. When these components are combined intentionally, your body is able to use food more efficiently, keeping energy levels steady throughout the day. Your body will always give feedback. If you feel sluggish after eating or hungry shortly after a meal, something may need adjusting, either the portion, the balance, or both. Many people eat "healthy" foods, but still do not feel well because there is no structure. Portion balance provides that structure, allowing your body to function the way it is designed to.

"It's not about eating less, it's about eating in a way that supports you."

Supplements: Support, Not the Foundation

Supplements can be helpful, but they are not the foundation of health. The body functions best when nutrients come from real, whole foods. Supplements are meant to fill gaps, not replace meals. Vitamins and minerals influence everything from energy and skin health to hormones and immune function, and when levels are low, the body will often signal it. However, whole foods offer something supplements cannot. They provide a complex network of nutrients, fiber, fats, and bioactive compounds that work together in ways isolated supplements cannot replicate.

Used thoughtfully, supplements can provide additional support. But more is not better. Overuse or random supplementation can create imbalances rather than correct them. The true foundation is consistency, daily habits that nourish the body over time.

Supplements can support you, but your habits are what truly shape your health.

Foods That Can Disrupt Hormonal Balance

Certain dietary patterns can quietly disrupt this balance over time. Diets high in heavily processed foods, excess sugar, refined carbohydrates, and unhealthy fats can contribute to inflammation and unstable blood sugar. Excess alcohol intake may also interfere with hormone regulation. At the same time, restrictions can be just as disruptive. Diets too low in fiber or healthy fats can limit the body's ability to produce and regulate hormones effectively. Hormones depend on nourishment, not deprivation. Healthy fats, in particular, play a powerful role.

They are essential building blocks for hormone production. Foods such as avocados, olive oil, wild-caught salmon, walnuts, flaxseed, chia seeds, and hemp seeds support this process. Hemp seeds, for example, are rich in gamma-linolenic acid (GLA), which may help support progesterone balance (Swanson et al., 2012). Beyond hormone production, these fats support brain function, mood stability, metabolic health, and inflammation regulation. When included consistently and intentionally, they help create the internal environment hormones need to function optimally. Hydration and electrolyte balance also matter. Sodium, when consumed in appropriate amounts, supports nerve signaling, fluid balance, and muscle function. While options like Himalayan pink salt contain trace minerals, their benefits should be viewed as supportive rather than transformative.

Equally important is the type of fat consumed. Diets high in omega-6–rich oils (such as sunflower, corn, soybean, and canola oils), particularly from processed foods, may contribute to inflammation when consumed in excess (Simopoulos, 2016). The issue is not omega-6 itself, but the imbalance commonly seen in modern diets. Shifting toward anti-inflammatory fats, such as olive oil, avocado oil, nuts, seeds, and fatty fish, helps restore that balance.

A hormone-supportive way of eating centers on whole, nutrient-dense foods:

- ♥ Colorful fruits and vegetables for antioxidants

- ♥ Whole grains for fiber and blood sugar stability

- ♥ Lean proteins for repair and sustained energy

- ♥ Healthy fats for hormone production and inflammation regulation

Chronic inflammation can quietly contribute to fatigue, metabolic issues, cardiovascular risk, and hormone imbalance. Supporting the body through consistent, anti-inflammatory nutrition is not about perfection, it is about creating sustainable patterns that promote long-term balance. This way of eating is nourishment, not restriction.

Getting P(her)sonal Recipes: Protein Balance Bowl

Ingredients:

- ♥ 1 cup of cooked quinoa or brown rice

- ♥ ½ cup roasted sweet potato

- ♥ 1 cup sautéed spinach or kale

- ♥ 1 protein: grilled salmon, chicken, or chickpeas

- ♥ ½ avocado

- ♥ 1 tbsp pumpkin seeds

- ♥ 1 tbsp olive oil

- ♥ Lemon, garlic, and pink salt (to taste)

Why this works:

This meal is designed to support stable blood sugar, hormone production, and sustained energy. It combines protein, fiber, and healthy fats to help regulate appetite, support metabolic function, and reduce energy crashes throughout the day.

Herbs That Support Hormone Balance:

- ♥ Ashwagandha – supports stress regulation and cortisol balance

- ♥ Maca – supports energy, mood, and hormonal rhythm

- ♥ Red clover – may support estrogen balance

- ♥ Black cohosh – often used for menopausal symptoms

- ♥ Spearmint tea – may help with androgen balance (great for acne/PCOS)

Herbs can be used in teas, powders, or supplements depending on your needs.

Through balanced meals, gut support, stable blood sugar, nourishing fats, and thoughtful lifestyle choices, you begin to shape hormonal harmony from within.

Big Sister Summary: The Science Behind It

Sis, everything we've talked about in this chapter isn't just "wellness talk," it's grounded in real science. Hormonal symptoms like mood swings, irregular cycles, weight changes, fatigue, and skin issues are often linked to imbalances in estrogen, progesterone, testosterone, insulin, and cortisol (Rosenfield, 2020; Santoro et al., 2021). And one of the most powerful ways to influence these hormones is through how you nourish your body. Research shows that eating regular, balanced meals helps stabilize insulin and cortisol levels, which can improve energy, mood, and menstrual patterns (Jakubowicz et al., 2015). Whole, nutrient-dense foods, especially those rich in plants, support blood sugar regulation, reduce inflammation, and improve overall metabolic health (Aune et al., 2017). Your gut plays a major role, too. The gut microbiome directly influences estrogen metabolism, inflammation, thyroid function, and even stress responses through the gut-brain axis (Baker et al., 2019; Thursby & Juge, 2017). This is why fiber, prebiotics, and probiotics matter more than most people realize. Blood sugar stability is another key piece. Meals that combine protein, fiber, and healthy fats help prevent glucose spikes that can disrupt mood, sleep, and energy (Ludwig et al., 2018). And healthy fats themselves are essential, omega-3 fatty acids support hormone production and reduce inflammation (Swanson et al., 2012), while excessive intake of processed oils may increase inflammatory responses (Simopoulos, 2016). Even certain herbs, like ashwagandha, maca, and ginseng, have been studied for their potential to support stress regulation and overall hormonal balance (Lopresti et al., 2019; Brooal, 2019). So no, you're not imagining things. Your body is responding exactly as it was designed to. When you nourish it with intention, it responds with balance.

I'm just here to guide you through it, like a big sister who reads the research first.

Pause & Reflect

No pressure, just awareness.

"If your body could rate how supported it feels by the way you're eating right now... what would it say?"

Getting P(her)sonal

A Self-Development Guide

Getting P(her)sonal

A Self-Development Guide

Getting P(her)sonal

A Self-Development Guide

Getting P(her)sonal

A Self-Development Guide

Getting P(her)sonal

A Self-Development Guide

Getting P(her)sonal

A Self-Development Guide

Getting P(her)sonal

A Self-Development Guide

Getting P(her)sonal
A Self-Development Guide

Getting P(her)sonal

A Self-Development Guide

Block 4: Stress & Hormone Connection

How Stress Affects Cortisol & Hormones

Stress has a way of quietly shaping how we think, feel, and even how our hormones respond. While stress is a natural part of being human, understanding how it works gives us the ability to soften its impact and return to balance with more intention.

When the body senses stress, hormones like cortisol and adrenaline increase to protect you. While helpful short-term, chronic stress can disrupt hormone balance, affecting mood, sleep, digestion, and energy. Over time, persistent stress can affect mood, metabolism, sleep, skin health, and digestion, ultimately interfering with hormonal balance (Chrousos, 2009). What may feel like "random anxiety" is often the body communicating underlying imbalances, whether related to blood sugar instability, gut health, nutrient deficiencies, excessive caffeine intake, or emotional overload. These signals are not random; they are meaningful.

Anxiety, Worry & Low Self-Esteem

Anxiety rarely appears without context. It is often the result of multiple factors coming together, hormonal shifts, digestive imbalance, nutrient gaps, emotional stress, or even unresolved experiences resurfacing in subtle ways. When these layers build, the body begins to express what it cannot ignore. Anxiety can make every day experiences feel heavier, more intense, and harder to navigate. But there is something important to remember: anxiety is responsive. When the body is supported, it often begins to soften.

Small, consistent shifts can make a meaningful difference:

- ♥ Increasing mineral intake through water and nutrient-dense foods

- ♥ Supporting the nervous system with magnesium (such as citrate or glycinate)

- ♥ Eating in a way that promotes stable blood sugar

- ♥ Maintaining a consistent and restorative sleep routine

- ♥ Seeking therapeutic support when needed

- ♥ Creating gentle, predictable daily rhythms

Stress Management Tools

The goal is not to eliminate stress; it is to build resilience. When the body feels supported, it becomes better equipped to move through stress without becoming overwhelmed.

Effective support often includes:

- ♥ Setting and maintaining healthy boundaries

- ♥ Practicing meditation or grounding techniques

- ♥ Creating consistent, calming routines

- ♥ Incorporating herbs and foods that support stress regulation

- ♥ Moving the body regularly and intentionally

Movement for Hormone Regulation

Movement, in particular, is one of the most powerful tools for regulating stress. Exercise helps balance cortisol levels, improve mood, and support overall hormone function (Hackney, 2006). Strength training is especially beneficial. It supports muscle tone and metabolic health and plays a key role in maintaining bone density over time (Guadalupe-Grau et al., 2009). As estrogen levels decline, maintaining bone density becomes increasingly important, making resistance and weight-bearing exercise essential for long-term health (Ader, 2007). This does not require intense or overwhelming workouts. Consistent, moderate strength training, even a few times per week, can create meaningful change. Practices like yoga offer additional benefits by combining movement with breath and stillness. This helps regulate the nervous system, shifting the body out of a constant "fight-or-flight" state. Mindfulness techniques, such as deep breathing, body scans, and slow meditation, further support this process by calming the system from within.

When Stress & Hormones Interact

Women often experience stress more intensely because our hormonal systems are naturally dynamic. As stress levels rise, they can disrupt the balance of estrogen and progesterone, leading to mood swings, fatigue, irregular cycles, cravings, sleep disturbances, and changes in weight. This is not a weakness; it is physiology.

When we begin to understand this connection, we can respond with more compassion rather than frustration. A holistic approach, one that includes movement, mindfulness, boundaries, nutrition, and emotional awareness, helps build resilience and supports the body's ability to regulate hormones more effectively.

Psychoneuroimmunology (Mind-Body Connection)

The field of psychoneuroimmunology explores how thoughts and emotions influence the immune and endocrine systems

(Ader, 2007). Its findings are both simple and powerful: Your body responds to what your mind repeatedly experiences. Through neuroplasticity, repeated thoughts shape neural pathways over time (Ader, 2007). Chronic worry or negative self-talk can activate stress hormones, while prolonged stress can suppress immune function, disrupt hormonal balance, and increase inflammation.

This is why stress often manifests physically:

- ♥ Fatigue

- ♥ Digestive discomfort

- ♥ Skin changes or breakouts

- ♥ Mood fluctuations

- ♥ Irregular menstrual cycles

But the same system that responds to stress can also respond to support.

Practices such as self-compassion, gratitude, deep breathing, and rest create measurable physiological shifts. They help regulate neurotransmitters like serotonin, dopamine, and oxytocin chemicals associated with calm, connection, and emotional stability (Hofmann, 2010). Every supportive thought becomes part of your healing environment.

Why This Matters for Women's Health

Because women's hormones follow cyclical patterns, they are particularly sensitive to emotional and psychological inputs (Baker & Driver, 2007). This means that mental and emotional practices are not optional; they are integral to physical health. Practices such as journaling, therapy, meditation, breathwork, and meaningful connection help regulate the nervous system and, in turn, influence hormonal balance. These tools work alongside nutrition and lifestyle habits, not separately from them. Your thoughts are not just passing experiences; they are signals. They influence the hormones that shape your mood, energy, metabolism, fertility, and even your skin. When you begin to cultivate a more supportive inner environment, you strengthen your body's ability to regulate, recover, and maintain balance over time. I didn't realize how much stress was affecting my body until I slowed down enough to notice the patterns. That awareness changed everything.

Big Sister Perspective: What the Science Confirms

Sis, the connection between stress and hormones is real and well supported by research. Chronic stress elevates cortisol levels, which can disrupt estrogen and progesterone balance, affect blood sugar regulation, and influence gut health, one of the central hubs of hormone regulation (Smith & Vale, 2006; Mayer et al., 2015). That's why symptoms like anxiety, fatigue, breakouts, and mood swings are not "all in your head." They are signals that your body is overwhelmed and asking for support. The encouraging part is that the body responds to care. Research shows that practices such as mindfulness, balanced nutrition, regular movement, and targeted nutrients like magnesium can help regulate the nervous system and support hormonal balance (Hofmann et al., 2010; Lopresti et al., 2019). You are not broken. Your body is responding exactly as it was designed to. And with the right support, it knows how to find its way back to balance.

Pause & Reflect

No pressure, answer freely and even journal!

"What has been weighing on you lately, and has your body been asking you to slow down in ways you've been trying to push past?"

Getting P(*her*)sonal

A Self-Development Guide

Getting P(her)sonal

A Self-Development Guide

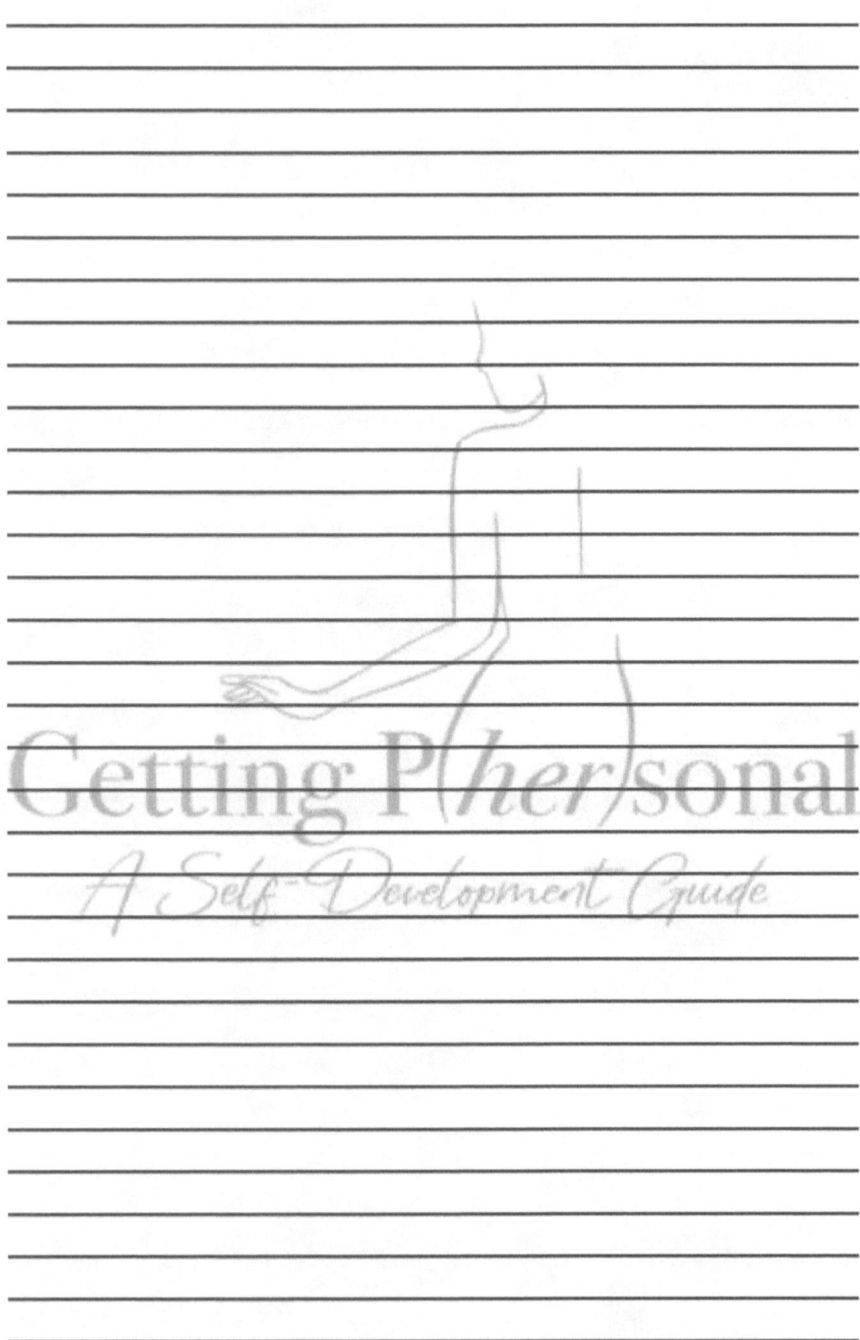

Getting P(her)sonal
A Self-Development Guide

Getting P(her)sonal

A Self-Development Guide

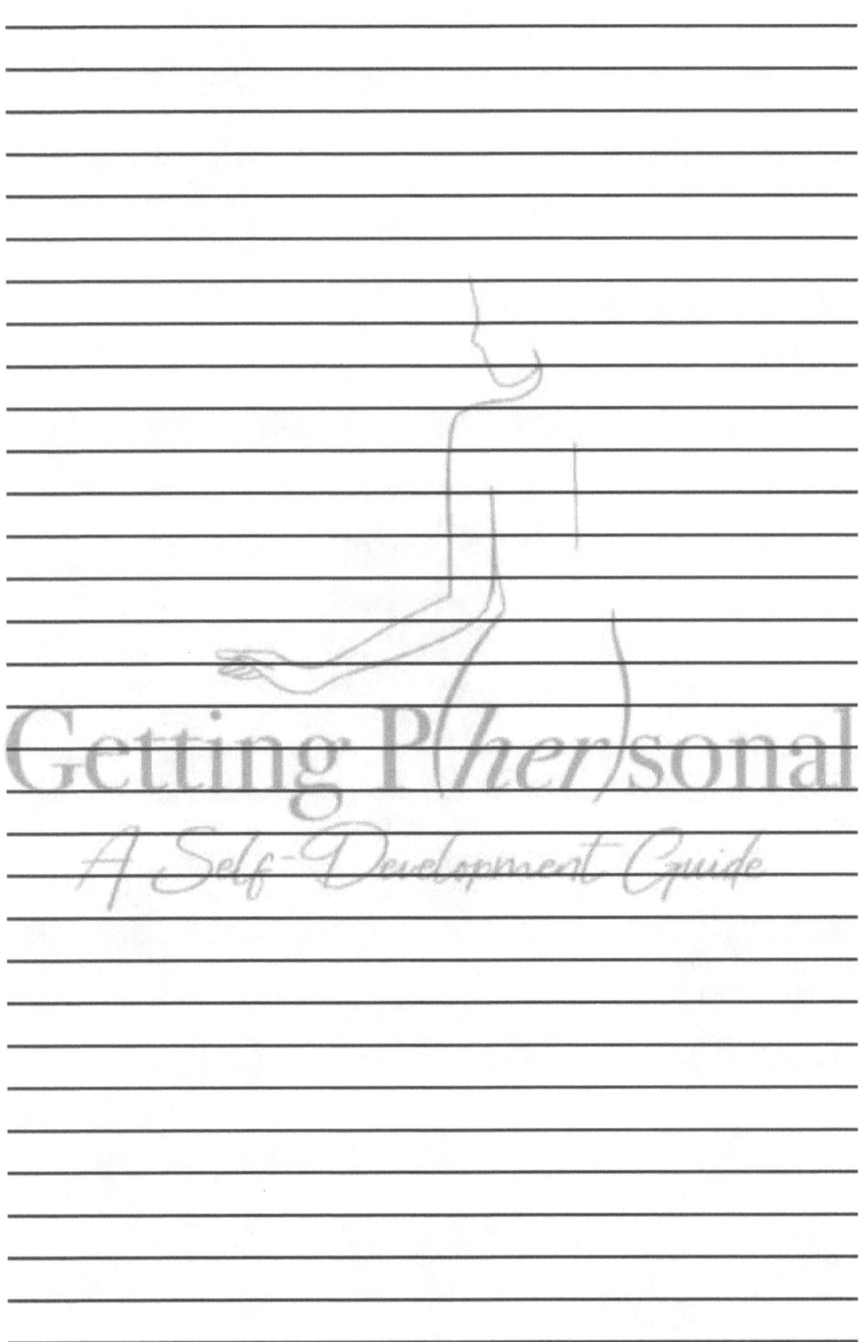
Getting P(her)sonal
A Self-Development Guide

Getting P(her)sonal
A Self-Development Guide

Getting P(her)sonal

A Self-Development Guide

Getting P(her)sonal

A Self-Development Guide

Getting P(*her*)sonal

A Self-Development Guide

Getting P(her)sonal

A Self-Development Guide

Getting P(her)sonal

A Self-Development Guide

Getting P(her)sonal

A Self-Development Guide

Getting P(her)sonal

A Self-Development Guide

Getting P(her)sonal

A Self-Development Guide

Block 5: The Power of Sleep

Listen, no matter who you are, what you do, or how many responsibilities you carry, you need sleep. We all do. Rest is not optional. It is the foundation your mental, emotional, and physical health is built on. You can show up for your work, your family, your goals, and your dreams, but without rest, you are trying to build a full life on an empty battery. Sleep is not just about closing your eyes. It is where your body does its most important behind-the-scenes work: repairing cells, regulating hormones, restoring your skin, supporting hair growth, processing memories, and resetting your emotional state (Walker, 2017). And no, five hours and a prayer will not sustain you. Most adults need around 7–9 hours of sleep each night to support optimal health, recovery, and overall functioning (Cappuccio et al., 2010). Even when that feels difficult, consistency matters more than perfection.

How Sleep Affects Hormones

Sleep is one of the strongest predictors of long-term health, and the research is clear. Poor sleep is associated with weakened immunity, weight changes, hormonal imbalance, mood disturbances, memory issues, inflammation, and increased risk of chronic conditions such as heart disease and diabetes (Cappuccio et al., 2010). But the opposite is just as powerful. When sleep is consistent and restorative, mental clarity improves, hormones stabilize, metabolism functions more efficiently, and emotional regulation becomes easier. Even your skin reflects that internal balance. When sleep is disrupted, the body begins to compensate. Late nights, whether from stress, work, scrolling, or overstimulation, create a ripple effect. Mornings feel heavier. Energy drops.

Motivation declines. And over time, this creates a cycle:

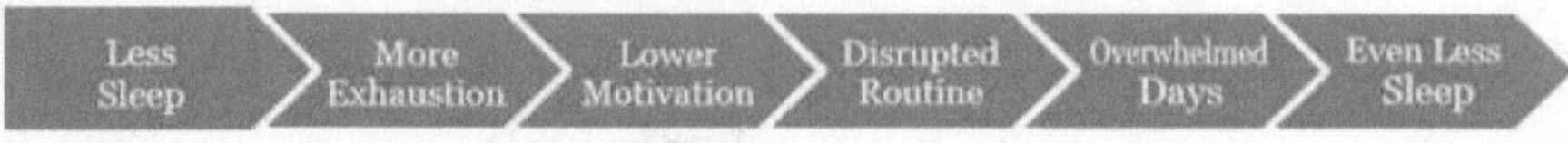

And just like that, the cycle continues, unless you intentionally break it.

Sleep, Self-Care & Emotional Boundaries

Sleep is essential for hormone regulation, cognitive function, and overall health. During sleep, your body repairs cells, regulates hormones, and restores energy systems. Your body needs consistency, regular sleep and wake times, darkness at night, reduced blue light exposure, and a calming evening routine. Protecting your sleep often means setting limits with work, creating space for yourself, stepping away from constant stimulation, and choosing routines that support your peace. These choices may seem small, but they communicate something powerful to your body: that rest is allowed. Self-care is not just what you do when you are overwhelmed; it is what prevents burnout in the first place. When you prioritize rest, your endocrine system responds. Cortisol levels begin to decrease, the nervous system settles, and emotional resilience strengthens. You feel more grounded, more present, and more like yourself.

Building a Sleep Rhythm That Supports You

Most people need 7–9 hours to fully recharge, but life can make that tricky (Cappuccio et al. 2010). When sleep gets cut short, the brain, especially the hippocampus, struggles to process memories, regulate emotions, and stay focused. That's why simple tasks feel harder, moods feel heavier, and mornings feel like climbing a mountain barefoot.

Sleep deprivation doesn't just leave you feeling tired; it affects how your entire body functions, including:

- ♥ Motivation and drive

- ♥ Decision-making and focus

- ♥ Stress tolerance

- ♥ Digestion and gut health

- ♥ Appetite regulation

- ♥ Hormonal balance

Everything in the body is connected.

Supporting your sleep does not require a complete lifestyle overhaul; it begins with small, consistent shifts. Creating a relaxing nighttime routine, reducing screen exposure, and keeping your sleep environment cool, dark, and calm can signal to your body that it is safe to rest. Going to bed at a similar time each night helps regulate your internal clock, while balanced meals throughout the day support hormone stability.

Gentle practices like journaling, stretching, breathwork, or light meditation can help release the mental and physical tension that builds over time. When needed, additional support, such as magnesium or mineral intake, can further support relaxation and nervous system regulation. These changes may seem small, but over time, they create meaningful shifts.

Little changes truly add up.

The Benefits of Restorative Sleep

When sleep becomes consistent and restorative, the effects are felt throughout the body. Skin appears clearer, the immune system strengthens, hormones regulate more smoothly, and moods become more stable. Focus sharpens, energy becomes more consistent, and inflammation begins to decrease. Sleep is not just rest; it is your body's most powerful recovery tool.

Sleep & Gut Health

Sleep and gut health are deeply interconnected. A well-rested body supports more efficient digestion and a balanced microbiome. While prebiotics, probiotics, yogurt, and fermented foods all play a role, sleep itself helps regulate inflammation and support beneficial gut bacteria (Irwin, 2015). Rest and gut health move together. When one improves, the other often follows.

Big Sister Reminder: Improving Your Sleep

You deserve to wake up feeling restored, not just functional. When you give your body the sleep it needs, everything else begins to feel more manageable: your mood, your motivation, your energy, and your overall sense of well-being.

Sis, sleep is not just "rest," it is biology, and the research is clear. Getting less than 7–9 hours disrupts hormone regulation, weakens immunity, and affects mood, memory, and even skin health (Walker, 2017; Irwin, 2015). Your body does its deepest healing at night—repairing cells, balancing cortisol, supporting metabolism, and resetting your emotional systems. Chronic sleep deprivation has been linked to increased risk of heart disease, weight changes, anxiety, and inflammation (Cappuccio et al., 2010). So when I tell you to prioritize sleep, it is not pressure, it is care. It is big sister love, backed by real evidence.

Pause & Reflect

Answer at your own pace!

**"Are you truly resting... or just pushing through
until your body forces you to stop?"**

Getting P(her)sonal

A Self-Development Guide

Getting P(her)sonal

A Self-Development Guide

Getting P(her)sonal

A Self-Development Guide

Getting P(her)sonal

A Self-Development Guide

Getting P(her)sonal

A Self-Development Guide

Getting P(her)sonal

A Self-Development Guide

Getting P(her)sonal

A Self-Development Guide

Getting P(her)sonal

A Self-Development Guide

Getting P(her)sonal

A Self-Development Guide

Getting P(her)sonal

A Self-Development Guide

Block 6: Advocacy & Self-Empowerment

Understanding Health Professionals

Sis, taking care of your health isn't something you have to do alone. Think of it as building your own personal support team. When life feels confusing, your body feels out of sync, or you simply need answers, there are professionals whose purpose is to guide you, support you, and help you feel grounded in your care.

Dietitians help you understand what your body actually needs, not what the internet says is trending this week. They guide you in building balanced meals, identifying nutritional gaps, and supporting concerns like hormonal imbalance, gut health, or chronic conditions. They also help you navigate resources and access to care, especially when the system feels overwhelming.

They make "food as medicine" feel realistic and sustainable. Your doctor and nurses help you see the bigger picture, how your systems, symptoms, and overall health connect. They focus on prevention, early detection, and medical guidance that goes beyond surface-level answers. They can connect you with specialists, testing, and long-term strategies that support your overall well-being. Think of them as your body's strategist. A therapist supports the part of you that isn't always visible, your thoughts, emotions, stress, healing, and growth. They help you understand patterns, build boundaries, process experiences, and develop emotional resilience. Mental and emotional health are deeply connected to hormonal health, and therapists play a key role in helping you feel balanced from the inside out.

Finding Balance When To Seek Support

When health professionals work together, your care becomes more complete. You are no longer guessing, you are making informed decisions with support.

You might consider reaching out for support when:

- ♥ Your symptoms feel persistent, confusing, or overwhelming

- ♥ You notice changes in your mood, energy, sleep, or cycle

- ♥ You feel dismissed, unheard, or unsure about your care

- ♥ You simply want guidance instead of figuring everything out alone.

And remember, asking for help is not a weakness. It is one of the strongest, most self-aware things you can do.

Advocating For Your Body

Sis, if there's one thing I want you to take from this entire guide, it's this: **you are your body's greatest advocate**. No one knows your symptoms, your cycles, your intuition, or your struggles better than you do. And as you move through all the hormonal changes life brings, puberty, postpartum, perimenopause, and menopause, you deserve care that listens, respects, and adapts to you. Hormonal shifts are powerful, and they touch every part of your life, from your mood and metabolism to your skin, sleep, and even your oral health. Yep, your hormones talk to your teeth too. That's why staying informed and speaking up about your needs is not being "difficult," it's being responsible, wise, and deeply connected to your own well-being. As you age and evolve, your healthcare journey should evolve with you. The most effective care is collaborative: you + your providers working together to honor your history, preferences, genetics, lifestyle, and goals. This is the heart of personalized, preventive, patient-centered healthcare... and you deserve nothing less. Stress, nutrition, sleep, and emotional health all play their part, too. The more you understand the signs your body sends you, even the confusing ones, the better equipped you'll be to ask for the support you need. And sometimes that support comes from medication, sometimes from lifestyle changes, sometimes from therapy, herbs, or nutrition. There is no "one right way," there is only your way, shaped lovingly and thoughtfully over time.

Advocating for yourself doesn't have to be loud or confrontational, it can be clear, calm, and confident. You can start by:

- Coming prepared with your symptoms, questions, or concerns written down

- Asking for clarification if something doesn't make sense

- Requesting testing, referrals, or second opinions when needed

- Speaking up if you feel dismissed or unheard

- Taking notes or bringing someone you trust to appointments

- Trusting your intuition, if something feels off, it deserves attention

You are not asking for too much. You are asking for care.

Research consistently shows that patient engagement and self-advocacy are linked to better health outcomes, improved satisfaction with care, and more accurate diagnoses. I created this guide for women like us, women who've felt overwhelmed, unheard, or lost in medical jargon...women who needed a starting point, a safe space, and a community that would walk with them through the journey instead of telling them to "just figure it out."

So, here's your reminder:

- ♥ You are not alone.

- ♥ You are allowed to ask questions.

- ♥ You are allowed to take up space in the exam room.

- ♥ You are allowed to choose the path that feels right for your body. This is your new community, the one that cares about your wellness, celebrates your progress, and wants to hear every chapter of your story.

We've got you, sis.

And from here on out, I hope you've got you, too.

Pause & Reflect

This is your reminder; you have a voice here.

**"If you fully trusted yourself as your body's advocate...
what would you start speaking up about today?"**

Getting P(her)sonal

A Self-Development Guide

Getting P(her)sonal
A Self-Development Guide

Getting P(her)sonal

A Self-Development Guide

Getting P(her)sonal

A Self-Development Guide

Getting Phersonal

A Self-Development Guide

Getting P(her)sonal

A Self-Development Guide

Getting P(her)sonal

A Self-Development Guide

Getting P(her)sonal

A Self-Development Guide

Getting P(her)sonal

A Self-Development Guide

Getting P(*her*)sonal

A Self-Development Guide

Getting P(her)sonal

A Self-Development Guide

Getting P(her)sonal

A Self-Development Guide

Getting P(her)sonal

A Self-Development Guide

MUNA'S FAVES COOKING CORNER

Your space to nourish, explore, and create

Sis, this is your cozy corner.
A space where nourishment meets intention, where you can support your hormones through food, explore new recipes, and make each meal your own. Think of this as your personal kitchen journal, guided by balance, nourishment, and a little big-sister wisdom.

About this cooking corner...

This section is designed to support you through every season of hormonal change, whether that's PMS, postpartum, perimenopause, menopause, or simply wanting to feel more balanced in your everyday life.

What This Section Supports:

- ♥ Simple, hormone-friendly nutrition guidance

- ♥ Practical ways to use herbs, spices, and balanced cooking methods

- ♥ Easy, adaptable recipes for everyday life

- ♥ Building meals that support hormone health without overwhelm

- ♥ Space for you to create and personalize your own recipes

How Food Supports Your Hormones

Hormones thrive on consistency, steady blood sugar, balanced meals, and the right combination of fats, protein, and micronutrients.

- ♥ steadier energy

- ♥ clearer skin

- ♥ more balanced moods

- ♥ improved sleep

- ♥ more regulated cycles

- ♥ reduced bloating

- ♥ lower inflammation

The meals in this section are designed to make hormone-supportive eating feel simple, approachable, and sustainable.

Breakfast

Because how you start your day sets the tone for your hormones. A balanced breakfast helps regulate blood sugar, support metabolism, and stabilize mood for the rest of the day.

Make-Ahead Oatmeal (Steel-cut or rolled oats)

Ingredients

- ♥ 3 cups oats
- ♥ 6 cups water
- ♥ 2–4 tbsp ground flax
- ♥ ½ tsp salt
- ♥ ½ tsp nutmeg
- ♥ ½ tsp cinnamon
- ♥ 2 tbsp coconut oil
- ♥ Maple syrup (optional)

Directions:

1. Bring the water and salt to a gentle boil in a medium saucepan.
2. Add the oats, reduce heat to low, and let simmer for 5–10 minutes, stirring occasionally until slightly thickened.

3. Stir in the ground flax and mix well to combine.

4. Remove from heat, allow to cool slightly, then transfer to a container and refrigerate overnight.

5. The next morning, reheat on the stovetop or in the microwave, adding a splash of water or milk if needed to loosen the texture.

6. Stir in cinnamon, nutmeg, coconut oil, and maple syrup to taste before serving.

Optional: Add Greek yogurt for extra protein and balance.

<u>Feta Avocado Toast</u>

A simple, satisfying combination of healthy fats, fiber, and protein, perfect for steady energy and hormone support.

Ingredients:

- ♥ 1–2 slices whole-grain bread
- ♥ ½ ripe avocado
- ♥ 1–2 tsp fresh lemon juice
- ♥ Salt and black pepper, to taste
- ♥ 2–3 tbsp crumbled feta cheese

Optional: fresh basil, cilantro, chili flakes, or drizzle of olive oil

Directions:

1. Toast the whole-grain bread to your desired level of crispness.

2. In a small bowl, mash the avocado with lemon juice, salt, and pepper until smooth but slightly textured.

3. Spread the avocado mixture evenly over the toast.

4. Top with crumbled feta cheese.

5. Add optional toppings like herbs, chili flakes, or a light drizzle of olive oil.

6. Serve immediately and enjoy.

Why This Works

- Healthy fats (avocado): support hormone production and satiety

- Fiber (whole-grain bread): helps regulate blood sugar

- Protein (feta): supports sustained energy and fullness

Lunch

Midday meals that keep your energy stable and your body supported

Garlic Chicken & Mint Lettuce Wraps

Light, refreshing, and protein-rich, perfect for supporting stable energy and balanced hormones.

Ingredients:

- 1 lb ground or finely minced chicken
- 3 cloves garlic, minced
- 1 tbsp olive oil or avocado oil
- 1–2 tbsp fresh mint, finely chopped
- 1 tbsp fresh cilantro (optional)
- 1 tbsp low-sodium soy sauce or coconut aminos
- 1 tsp sesame oil (optional, for flavor)

- ½ tsp ground ginger (or 1 tsp fresh grated ginger)
- Salt and black pepper, to taste
- 1 head butter lettuce or romaine leaves (washed and separated)

Optional toppings: shredded carrots, sliced cucumber, green onions, chili flakes, or lime wedges

Directions:

1. Heat olive oil in a pan over medium heat.

2. Add minced garlic and sauté for about 30 seconds until fragrant (do not burn).

3. Add the ground chicken and cook for 5–7 minutes, breaking it apart as it browns.

4. Stir in soy sauce (or coconut aminos), ginger, sesame oil, salt, and pepper. Cook for another 2–3 minutes until fully combined and cooked through.

5. Remove from heat and gently mix in fresh mint and cilantro.

6. Spoon the warm chicken mixture into lettuce cups.

7. Add optional toppings like carrots, cucumber, or a squeeze of lime for extra freshness.

8. Fold and enjoy immediately.

Why This Works

- ♥ Lean protein (chicken): Supports stable blood sugar and helps reduce cravings while providing key building blocks for hormone health

- ♥ Healthy fats (olive or avocado oil): Support hormone regulation, brain function, and nutrient absorption

- ♥ Fresh herbs (mint & cilantro): Provide antioxidants and support digestion

- ♥ Low-glycemic base (lettuce wraps): Helps prevent blood sugar spikes and energy crashes

- ♥ Ginger & garlic: Support inflammation balance and overall metabolic health

Sautéed Kale with Kumquats (Served Chilled)

A bright, nutrient-rich dish that supports digestion and adds a refreshing balance of citrus and greens.

Ingredients:

- ♥ 1 bunch kale, stems removed and leaves chopped
- ♥ 1–2 kumquats, thinly sliced (seeds removed)
- ♥ 2 tbsp olive oil
- ♥ 1–2 cloves garlic, minced
- ♥ ½ tbsp lemon juice
- ♥ Salt and black pepper, to taste

Optional: pinch of red pepper flakes or drizzle of honey

Directions:

1. Heat olive oil in a pan over medium heat.

2. Add garlic and sauté until fragrant, about 30 seconds.

3. Add chopped kale and sauté for 4–6 minutes, stirring occasionally, until softened but still vibrant.

4. Add sliced kumquats and cook for another 1–2 minutes to release their natural citrus flavor.

5. Season with salt, pepper, and optional lemon juice or red pepper flakes.

6. Remove from heat and allow to cool slightly.

7. Serve chilled or at room temperature.

Why This Works

- Leafy greens (kale): support liver function and hormone metabolism

- Citrus (kumquats): provide antioxidants and support digestion

- Healthy fats (olive oil): support nutrient absorption and hormone production

Dinner

Balanced meals to nourish your body, support recovery, and promote hormonal stability.

Mango Salsa Salmon with Rice and Broccoli

Fresh, vibrant, and rich in anti-inflammatory nutrients, this meal combines healthy fats, fiber, and protein to support hormone balance and steady energy.

Ingredients:

- 2 salmon fillets
- 1 tbsp olive oil
- Salt and black pepper, to taste
- ½ tsp garlic powder
- ½ tsp paprika or dried herbs (optional)

Mango Salsa:

- 1 ripe mango, diced
- 2 tbsp red onion, finely chopped
- 1 small jalapeño, finely chopped (optional)
- 2 tbsp fresh cilantro, chopped
- Juice of 1 lime
- 1 tbsp olive oil
- Pinch of salt

For Serving:

- Steamed broccoli
- White or brown rice

Directions

1. Preheat a grill pan or skillet over medium heat.

2. Drizzle salmon with olive oil and season with salt, pepper, and spices.

3. Cook salmon for 4–6 minutes per side, or until flaky and fully cooked.

4. In a bowl, combine mango, onion, jalapeño, cilantro, lime juice, olive oil, and salt. Mix gently.

5. Plate salmon with rice and steamed broccoli.

6. Spoon mango salsa over the salmon and serve immediately.

Why This Works

- ♥ Omega-3 fats (salmon): reduce inflammation and support hormone production

- ♥ Fiber (broccoli + rice): supports digestion and blood sugar balance

- ♥ Antioxidants (mango, herbs): help reduce oxidative stress

Snacks

Simple, nourishing options to keep your energy steady between meals. Balanced snacks help prevent blood sugar dips and support consistent energy throughout the day.

- ♥ Cottage cheese with blueberries

- ♥ Papaya and apple fruit salad

- ♥ Celery and carrots with hummus

Desserts

Yes, sis, dessert can absolutely be part of a balanced lifestyle.

The key is choosing options that include nutrients, healthy fats, and natural sweetness.

♥ Cherries dipped in dark chocolate

♥ Raspberries with coconut cream or Greek yogurt

♥ Cocoa chia pudding (rich in fiber and omega-3s)

Closing Message

Balance isn't about cutting things out; it's about building meals that truly support you. You can enjoy your food and nourish your body at the same time. When your meals include protein, fiber, and healthy fats, your body responds with more stable energy, fewer cravings, and a greater sense of overall well-being.

By filling your plate with whole, colorful, nutrient- dense foods, you're not just "eating healthy," you're supporting your hormones, your energy, your sleep, your skin, your gut, and your joy. And remember, this guide is not a rulebook. These are meals and practices that have helped me thrive, but your journey is your own. Add your favorite flavors, swap ingredients, explore new spices, make it yours. Your body will always tell you what it needs. Your job is to listen, stay curious, and care for yourself with intention and love.

Pause & Create

This is your space, make it yours.

**"If your body could design its perfect meal today...
what would be on your plate?"**

"What's one new ingredient, flavor, or recipe you've been curious to try for your body?"

"What meals make you feel the most nourished, energized, and like yourself?"

Getting P(*her*)sonal

A Self-Development Guide

Getting P(her)sonal

A Self-Development Guide

Getting P(her)sonal

A Self-Development Guide

Getting P(her)sonal

A Self-Development Guide

Getting P(*her*)sonal

A Self-Development Guide

Getting P(her)sonal

A Self-Development Guide

Getting P(her)sonal

A Self-Development Guide

Getting P(her)sonal

A Self-Development Guide

Getting P(her)sonal

A Self-Development Guide

Getting P(her)sonal

A Self-Development Guide

Getting P(*her*)sonal

A Self-Development Guide

Getting P(*her*)sonal

A Self-Development Guide

Getting P(her)sonal

A Self-Development Guide

Getting P(her)sonal

A Self-Development Guide

References.

Hormones, Endocrine Function & Reproductive Health

Aune, D., Chan, D., Greenwood, D. C., & Vieira, A. R. (2017). Fruit and vegetable intake and risk of chronic disease. International Journal of Epidemiology.

Baker, F. C., & Driver, H. S. (2007). Circadian rhythms, sleep, and the menstrual cycle. Sleep Medicine.

Chrousos, G. P. (2009). Stress and disorders of the stress system. Nature Reviews Endocrinology.

Diamanti-Kandarakis, E., & Dunaif, A. (2009). Insulin resistance and PCOS pathophysiology. Endocrine Reviews.

Guadalupe-Grau, A., Fuentes, T., Guerra, B., & Calbet, J. A. L. (2009). Exercise and bone mass in adults. Sports Medicine.

Hall, J. E., & Hall, M. E. (2021). Guyton and Hall textbook of medical physiology.

Leproult, R., & Van Cauter, E. (2010). Role of sleep and circadian rhythms in endocrine function. Endocrine Development.

Loucks, A. B. (2004). Energy availability and reproductive function in women. Exercise and Sport Sciences Reviews.

Ludwig, D. S., & Willett, W. (2018). The carbohydrate-insulin model and metabolic health. JAMA Internal Medicine.

Riggs, B. L., Khosla, S., & Melton, L. J. (2002). Sex steroids and the construction and conservation of the adult skeleton. Endocrine Reviews.

Santoro, N., & Azziz, R. (2021). Menopause and metabolic changes. Endocrine Reviews.

Jakubowicz, D., Froy, O., Wainstein, J., & Boaz, M. (2015). High-energy breakfast improves weight loss and hormonal regulation. Obesity.

Gut Health, Nutrition & Metabolism

Ader, R. (2007). Psychoneuroimmunology. Current Directions in Psychological Science.

Gibson, G. R., Hutkins, R., Sanders, M. E., & Prescott, S. L. (2017). The concept of prebiotics. Nature Reviews Gastroenterology.

Hackney, A. C. (2006). Exercise as a stressor to the human neuroendocrine system. CNS & Neurological Disorders.

Hofmann, S. G., Sawyer, A. T., Witt, A. A., & Oh, D. (2010). The effect of mindfulness-based therapy on anxiety and depression. Journal of Consulting and Clinical Psychology.

Mayer, E. A., Tillisch, K., & Gupta, A. (2015). Gut/brain axis and the microbiota. Journal of Clinical Investigation.

Mullur, R., Liu, Y. Y., & Brent, G. A. (2014). Thyroid hormone regulation of metabolism. Physiological Reviews.

Phillips, S. M. (2014). Protein requirements and muscle health. Applied Physiology, Nutrition, and Metabolism.

Rosenfield, R. L. (2020). Hormonal imbalance and endocrine disorders. Endocrine Reviews,

Simopoulos, A. P. (2016). Omega-6/omega-3 balance in health and disease. Biomedicine & Pharmacotherapy.

Swanson, D., Block, R., & Mousa, S. A. (2012). Omega-3 fatty acids in health and disease. Advances in Nutrition.

Thursby, E., & Juge, N. (2017). Introduction to the human gut microbiota. Biochemical Journal.

Zimmermann, M. B., & Kohrle, J. (2002). Selenium and thyroid function. Endocrine Reviews.

Stress, Brain, and Mind-Body Connection
Ader, R. (2007). Psychoneuroimmunology. Current Directions in Psychological Science.

Cappuccio, F. P., D'Elia, L., Strazzullo, P., & Miller, M. A. (2010). Quantity and quality of sleep and incidence of type 2 diabetes and cardiovascular disease. Diabetes Care.

Lopresti, A. L., Jacka, F. N., & Loughman, A. (2019). Adaptogens and stress response. Journal of Alternative and Complementary Medicine.

Smith, S. M., & Vale, W. W. (2006). The role of the hypothalamic-pituitary-adrenal axis in stress responses. Endocrine Reviews.

Sleep & Recovery
Benedict, C., Rønn, M. H., Tjener, K., & Hallschmid, M. (2016). Acute sleep deprivation alters gut microbiota. Molecular Metabolism.

Irwin, M. R. (2015). Why sleep is important for health: A psychoneuroimmunology perspective. Annual Review of Psychology.

Walker, M. (2017). Why we sleep: Unlocking the power of sleep and dreams. Scribner.

About the Author

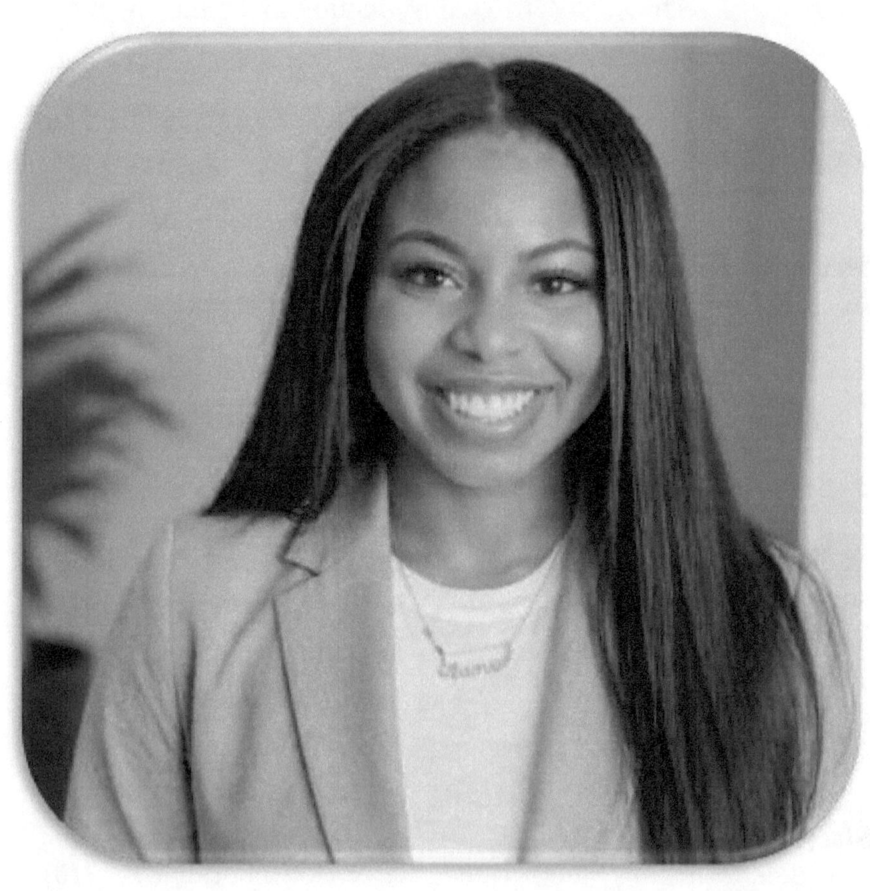

Muna Yvette Ezumah-Ezekwo

Bio

Muna Ezumah-Ezekwo is a public health researcher, educator, and wellness advocate deeply committed to helping women reconnect with their bodies in a way that feels supportive, intuitive, and never overwhelming. Her work blends science with compassion, offering guidance that is both evidence-based and deeply human.

She is driven by a commitment to truly understanding women's health beyond surface-level answers. Instead of quick fixes, she asks deeper questions and centers the real, lived experiences of women navigating their bodies every day. So many women are trying to care for themselves without ever being taught how. Instead of clarity, they are met with confusion, pressure, and one-size-fits-all advice. Muna knows this experience personally, which led her to create a space where women can explore their questions, share their experiences, and feel genuinely supported. Her work is rooted in a holistic, personal approach, one that helps women feel seen, heard, and empowered. Through her writing, Muna serves as both a guide and an advocate, helping women build clarity, confidence, and self-trust. She invites women to slow down, listen inward, and reconnect with their bodies in a deeper, more intentional way.

She believes healing is not about perfection, but about consistency, self-awareness, and giving yourself the care you deserve.

At the core of her message is a simple truth: your body is not working against you, it is always working for you.